MW00942249

The Anti-Inflammatory Diet

The Complete Anti-Inflammatory Diet Guide And Recipe Plan To Heal Inflammation, Reduce Pain, And Restore Health

Introduction

I want to thank you for purchasing this book, *"The Anti-Inflammatory Diet: The Complete Anti Inflammatory Diet Guide And Recipe Plan To Heal Inflammation, Reduce Pain, And Restore Overall Health"*.

This book contains a full outline of how to reduce bodily inflammation through implementing a diet that specifically targets anti-inflammatory foods. This reduction in inflammation not only improves existing health, but it also helps to ward off future conditions as well.

We will examine what inflammation actually is and identify those illnesses in which inflammation plays a significant role. We will then consider how dietary alterations can have a significant positive impact on healing, by identifying the foods and nutrients that should be consumed, together with those that should be avoided. This book will also provide a 7 day meal plan with delicious recipes for breakfast, lunch, and dinner.

Table of Contents

Chapter 1: What is Inflammation?

Before we begin to take a look at the anti-inflammatory diet and how it affects your body, it is important that we understand what inflammation actually is. In this chapter we are going to look at just that! Thereafter, we will source the food types and dietary plan necessary to help restore healing and overall wellbeing.

The Process of Inflammation

Most of us recognize inflammation as the swelling and redness most often associated with infection. However, it is important to note that inflammation does not have to be solely associated with infection. Nor does it even have to be visible on the outside of the body. Inflammation can be present on both the inside and outside of the body and can manifest itself as a result of many factors.

So what exactly happens when something on or in our bodies becomes inflamed? Inflammation is a natural response put into motion as an attempt by the body to protect itself. When the body notices something foreign or harmful present, the immune system then responds in an attempt to actually protect the body from that specific threat or attack. This response involves immune cells releasing inflammatory mediators such as histamine. The job of inflammatory mediators is to expand narrow blood vessels so that there is an increased blood flow to the area of irritation. This increased flow of blood also transports more of the inflammatory mediators to the site of injury or irritation. This response can then cause the heat and redness that we often see in injuries.

In addition to increasing blood flow to the affected area, inflammatory mediators also allow for more permeability of the narrow blood vessels. This means that more defense cells can pass through to the tissue of the affected area. When these defense cells then enter the infected area they bring along with them fluid which causes more inflammation to the injured area. This is what causes the swelling that we often refer to as inflammation.

These inflammatory mediators are not the only cause of extra fluid in the affected area. In addition, mucous membranes also release more excess fluid. This is put in motion so that the body can try to flush out the bacteria, foreign objects, or other sources of the inflammation causing the response.

Inflammation also helps the body to get rid of any dead cells in the area. This occurs as white cells are carried to the locus in question and they consume the dead cells, as well as the toxins present. The inflammatory process also repairs any tissues that have been damaged through injury or infection. The defense cells that are transported to the area of inflammation are quite short lived and die off. Ultimately, inflammation is reduced when the body no longer sees a need to continue transporting defense cells to the area. The inflammatory process can also be stopped through the use of medications which block the release of inflammation causing cells.

What Causes Chronic Inflammation?

So now that we have a better understanding of the inflammation process in general, let's take a look at what happens when things go awry. Chronic inflammation is a term used to refer to persistent inflammation that does not resolve. This lack of resolution can be the result of the toxin or invasive agent not being treated or due to a glitch in the body's autoimmune system. When chronic inflammation exists, the tissues of the body are not able to recover. This results in a wide range of symptoms which we will discuss shortly.

So what is it that causes the immune system to turn on the body to inflame and attack healthy tissues? While there has been wide ranging research into autoimmune disorders and various theories put forward, ultimately what causes the immune system to malfunction in this way is not fully known.

How Can We Treat What We Don't Understand?

While we don't know what causes chronic inflammation, we can treat existing inflammation and help to prevent future problems simply by eliminating contributing factors. One very important way to control inflammation is through diet. Diet can not only contribute to the cause of inflammation, but it can also make existing inflammation even worse.

Symptoms of Inflammatory Problems

There is a lot of variation in the diseases and illnesses that have inflammation as a symptom. Each of these has a variety of other symptoms accompanying them.

- Swelling – this is caused by the increase of fluid in the area as a result of the inflammatory mediators rushing to the affected point.

- Redness – Redness is caused by the dilation of small blood vessels by the immune system.

- Loss of function in the joints – Caused by inflammation that restricts movement of the joint.

- Joint pain – Caused by inflammation in the joint which makes it more difficult to move.

- Flu symptoms – Flu symptoms like fever, chills, stiffness of muscles, headache, and fatigue are the result of your body devoting energy to trying to eliminate a perceived toxin or invader. As your body diverts this energy to protecting itself, it diverts it away from "normal" functions leaving you feeling weak and drained.

- Other inflammatory symptoms are related to the conditions that cause the inflammation themselves. Symptoms related to the following conditions can also let you know that your body is fighting inflammation: heart disease, high blood pressure, ulcers, and irritable bowel syndrome.

Your doctor can test for inflammatory markers if you experience such symptoms. The inflammatory markers they may test for include:

- SED rate

- Elevated High Sensitivity C-Reactive Protein

- Elevated HDL

- Elevated blood glucose levels

- Elevated monocyte levels

- Elevated levels of ferritin

- Elevated levels of homocysteine

If any of these tests test positive, your doctor may order further tests based upon your current and previous health records. Your doctor may also suggest dietary changes to help regulate inflammation or treat inflammation of an unknown cause.

How is Inflammation Treated?

Treatment for acute inflammation is generally quite simple and involves identifying the source of infection or the wound. Once the problem has been identified it can be treated with antibiotics and regular wound cleaning. Once the infection is treated or the toxin has been removed, inflammation at the site will resolve because the body no longer needs to fight anything.

Treatment for chronic inflammation however, is more complex – particularly if the source is unknown. In many cases, treatment involves suppression of the body's immune system with steroids. While these drugs may reduce inflammation, they also tend to have a number of other undesired effects, since they can turn off the body's ability to protect itself. In some cases steroid treatment is unavoidable. Importantly however, some conditions can be successfully managed through other treatments such as diet. A simple change in diet to an anti-inflammatory plan can reduce inflammation and leave you feeling much healthier. This occurs because your body directly benefits from the anti-inflammatory properties of specific foods. Furthermore, your body also experiences decreased inflammation from a reduction of foods known to contribute to such symptoms.

Chapter 2: How Inflammation Plays in to Disease

In the previous chapter, we took a look at what inflammation is and what happens inside the body when inflammation happens. In this chapter we are going to take a closer look at some of the diseases that are associated with inflammation.

Joints and Inflammation

Perhaps one of the most recognized diseases when it comes to inflammation is arthritis. Arthritis is inflammation of the joints that not only causes pain, but that also causes stiffness and alters the range of motion. There are more than one hundred different types of arthritis, all of which are characterized by inflammation of the joints. The symptoms can vary in nature from mild, moderate to severe. They can be stable or may progressively get worse over time. There is also the potential for arthritis to impact organs within the body such as the kidneys, lungs and the heart.

The most common treatments for arthritis include non-steroidal anti-inflammatories, herbal supplementation, dietary change, and specialized medications.

Inflammation and Your Heart

Atherosclerosis – the buildup of fat inside the artery walls is characterized by chronic inflammation. When inflammation occurs in the circulatory system, it results in an increased chance of heart attack, stroke, and peripheral artery disease as arteries become narrower. This narrowing causes blood flow to significantly reduce. This then has a knock on affect in ensuring that oxygen flow to the bodily organs is also reduced.

The most common treatment for individuals with heart conditions is a drastic change in diet and exercise habits. Such changes have an overall positive impact on health, together with a reduction of inflammation.

Inflammation and Your Lungs

Inflammation in the lungs as well as other respiratory inflammation is a serious concern as it impacts breathing. When the airways become inflamed this is known as asthma. Asthma results in wheezing, inability to breath, tightness of the chest, shortness of breath, and coughing. Asthma can also result in death if symptoms are not controlled and treated. When the lungs become inflamed, this is most often known as pleurisy. Pleurisy is the inflammation of the lung tissue which causes pain and occurs as the lung tissues becoming irritated when they rub together. In addition to asthma and pleurisy, there are a number of other diseases that can cause lung inflammation. These include conditions such as sarcoidosis, lupus, and even rheumatoid arthritis.

Depending upon what is causing inflammation in the lungs and the respiratory system, treatments vary. For cases where inflammation is caused by bacteria, antibiotics can quickly remedy inflammation. For conditions such as asthma, lupus, sarcoidosis, and rheumatoid arthritis, treatment is palliative as there is no cure. Palliative treatment includes dietary change, exercise, and administration of other specialized drugs to control disease progress and prevent the auto-immune response.

Inflammation and Your Kidneys

Nephritis is the term used to refer to inflammation in the kidneys. Nephritis can result from toxins, infections and auto-immune disorders. Inflammation can take place within the kidneys and the structures inside them which leads to abdominal and back pain, urinary difficulties, and toxic buildup of elements in the body. When the kidneys become inflamed in these situations, they are unable to carry out their normal filtering functions or their function is partially compromised. Over time, the kidneys themselves can become damaged and can lead to permanent compromised kidney.

As with the lungs, treatment for kidney inflammation varies depending upon the cause of the inflammation. In the case where inflammation is caused by infection, anti-biotics are easily able to resolve the symptoms of inflammation and consequently eliminate it. In the case where kidney inflammation is caused by a more significant disease or illness, treatment is generally palliative and means assisting the kidneys through dialysis and treating other contributing factors to the disease in question. Diet is also a vital and necessary alteration for anyone with kidney affecting disease.

Inflammation and Auto-Immune Disorders

Almost all auto-immune disorders have inflammation as a symptom. This inflammation occurs because the body is attacking its own cells, tissues and fluids, mistaking them for invasive bodies. One way in which the body tries to flush out and destroy these invasive bodies (as we discussed above) is through inflammation. There are over 80 different auto-immune disorders and to date there are no specific cures. In order to eliminate an auto-immune disease it would be necessary to eliminate or reprogram the bodily immune system, and as of yet, this cannot be done. Some examples of auto-immune disorders that include inflammation as a symptoms include lupus, multiple sclerosis, rheumatoid arthritis, inflammatory bowel disease, and Hashimoto's disease. This is where diet can play such a vital role as the focus must be on relieving symptoms.

Inflammation and Neurological Disease

Inflammation has also been shown to play a role in neurological diseases. In diseases like multiple sclerosis, cells within the nervous system become hyper-activated and activate inflammatory responses by the body. This type of inflammation then contributes to progression of the disease itself. This means that controlling inflammation in neurological disease can help to slow down the disease progression.

Neurological disease, like many that we have already touched upon, are usually incurable. They can, however, be slowed down and moderated through disease modifying drugs and through controlling symptoms like inflammation. Disease modifying drugs are serious drugs in that they have significant effects on the body and contribute to a general feeling of illness. Treatment of symptoms however, can be assisted through the use of milder drugs like non-steroidal anti-biotics as well as through altering diet and exercise routines.

Inflammation and Cancer

Many people are not aware that inflammation plays a significant role in cancer. Inflammation within the body actually assists cancerous tumors in growing larger and spreading throughout the body. This occurs because as cancer cells grow and feed on nutrients in their environment, they release signals that draw immune cells to them. When these immune cells arrive on the scene, they enter cancerous cells and secrete cytokines which allow for the growth of blood vessels. These new blood vessels then provide more fuel to the cancer cells so that they can thrive and continue to grow.

We all know how aggressive treatment for cancer is, but often this treatment is also paired with dietary changes which help to control inflammation.

Chapter 3: The Anti-Inflammatory Diet

So now that we have covered the definition of inflammation and how inflammation plays in to various diseases, let's take a look at how it can be controlled through ones food intake. Dietary control is one of the easiest ways to regulate inflammation, without many of the side effects associated with regulating drugs.

What is the Anti-Inflammatory Diet?

Developed by Dr. Andrew Weil, the anti-inflammatory diet is designed not only to provide the body with fresh foods, but its main aim is to control, reduce and prevent inflammation within the body. Unlike many other diets that specifically target weight loss, although it can easily enable this, it is based predominantly on scientific knowledge of the nutrients within foods and their healing properties. Certain foods that many of us regularly consume increase the bodily inflammatory response, whereas other foods actually have anti-inflammatory properties which help to reduce and treat inflammation. The anti-inflammatory diet is designed with these food types in mind. Ultimately, this method works with the body to provide essential nutrients, while also bringing the body to a stable and healthy level of functioning.

What Are the Guidelines to the Anti-Inflammatory Diet?

We now need to examine the food types and nutrients that are essential to this diet plan.

Carbohydrates

When eating carbohydrates, focus on those that are made with whole grains and that do not contain sugar or wheat. Consume more foods like sweet potatoes and beans, eat pasta in moderation. Eliminate high fructose corn syrup. Avoid refined carbs such as sugar, white rice and bread. Such foods are a contributory factor to obesity and in turn increase inflammation within the body. On a diet of roughly 2000 calories a day a male should consume up to 300 grams of carbohydrates per day, while a women's intake should be about 200 grams.

Fats

When it comes to fats on the anti-inflammatory diet, make sure that you maintain a ratio of 1:2:1 of saturated: monosaturated: polysaturated fats. Cut your saturated fat levels down by eating less cheese, less fatty meats, less butter and cream, less high fat dairy, and eliminating or drastically reducing foodstuffs with palm kernel oil in them. Use extra virgin olive oil for cooking and simply avoid regular cooking oils, vegetable shortening, margarine, and foods with partially hydrogenated oils. Instead, focus on eating healthier fats like avocados, nuts, and nut based butters. You can also incorporate healthy fats by eating salmon, herring, and sardines in water. Hemp seeds and flax seeds are a wonderful source of essential fats together with omega/fish oil supplements.

Proteins

Make sure when consuming protein on the anti-inflammatory diet that you are catering your levels of protein intake to your health conditions. If you have a health condition that affects your liver or kidneys, ensure that you consume lower levels of protein. On the anti-inflammatory diet you also want to cut down the amount of animal proteins that you eat, although you can incorporate fish as well as natural yogurts and cheeses, and vegetable proteins. Whole-soy foods are a great source of protein on the anti-inflammatory diet. It is important to note that while soy can inhibit inflammation; if you have a sensitivity or allergy to such products it can result in having the opposite effect and should be avoided.

Fiber

Fiber is an important part of any diet and when adhering to the anti-inflammatory diet. You should strive to consume 40 grams of fiber each day. Your fiber intake can be provided through sources such as fresh vegetables, fruits, and whole grains. Cereal is also a great source for fiber, however, make sure to avoid sugary processed products and eat whole grain fibrous cereal instead.

Phytonutrients

Phytonutrients are a substance that are found in plants and play an important part in protecting against toxins and disease. Fruit and vegetables provide an abundance of Vitamin C, E, iron, and calcium which are all necessary for health, but they are also rich in phytonutrients. One should consume fruit and vegetables of all colors. Good examples are Kale, Spinach, Blueberries and Avocado. Make sure that these produce items are organic, or at least locally grown, and always cleanse them thoroughly before eating. Soy foods and cruciferous vegetables as well as dark chocolate (in moderation) are also great sources of phytonutrients. Tea and minimal red wine are also sources of phytonutrients as opposed to other alcohol and coffee.

Vitamins and Minerals

Once again, when it comes to vitamins and minerals, the best way to get your daily requirements is to include plenty of variety in fruits and vegetables in your diet. It is also beneficial to add an antioxidant vitamin to your daily routine and to take it with your main meal of the day. Dark leafy vegetables are a wonderful source of vitamins and minerals.

Supplements

Supplements may be necessary on the anti-inflammatory diet depending upon what you are eating. Most important is a fish oil supplement if you are not regularly eating fish as a part of your diet. In addition to fish oil, consider low-dose aspirin after talking to your doctor to see if it is right for you. Low-dose aspirin therapy helps your body to protect itself against inflammation. Depending upon your current level of health and other medications you may be taking, you may also benefit from the addition of anti-inflammatory herbs and supplements like devil's claw, ginger, or turmeric. Just be sure that you check any interactions between these supplements and your current treatments as well as make yourself aware of potential side effects of these supplements.

Beverages

Drink water. Drink plenty of water! Water helps to flush your body of toxins. Consequently it also reduces the inflammation that is caused by those very toxins. When you do drink water, ensure that it is filtered and has had potential contaminants removed from it. If you are not drinking water, focus on drinking tea, watered down fruit juices or naturally juiced vegetables and fruits. Avoid processed and preserved beverages like soft drinks and sports drinks.

What Foods Should Be Avoided on the Anti-Inflammatory Diet?

So, with these basic nutrient classes covered, what exactly should you be avoiding when you are following the anti-inflammatory diet? The following foods have an inflammatory causing effect.

- Foods that have high fructose content

- Foods with significant amounts of sugar

- Processed foods – if you can't pronounce an ingredient, it comes ready-made, or it comes packaged, chances are that it's processed.

- Excessive dairy

- Wheat, barley and rye – common inflammatory culprits.

- Gluten rich foods like seitan

- Peanuts

- Pre-mixed seasonings – these are high in artificial coloring as well as sugar and salt.

- Vegetable oil

- Red meat

- Trans-fat rich foods

- Processed corn

- Alcohol

- Processed meats

- Fried food

- Soda and energy drinks

- Grain fed meats

- Foods rich in additives and food additives like MSG

- Fast foods

- Large amounts of carbohydrates/starches

What Foods Can Be Eaten on the Anti-Inflammatory Diet?

Now that we have covered what you shouldn't eat on the anti-inflammatory diet, let's take a look at the foods that you should incorporate. Many of these foods are foods that have anti-inflammatory properties.

- Cruciferous (cabbage family) vegetables

- Berries - particularly blueberries and raspberries

- Garlic

- Wild salmon and other fresh fish

- Extra virgin olive oil

- Sweet potato

- Green tea

- Leafy greens

- Avocados

- Shiitake mushrooms

- Lean free range grass fed meats

- Eggs

- Fruits and vegetables – tomatoes, cherries and oranges contain excellent nutrients. Cinnamon is also well known for its anti-inflammatory benefits.

- Beans and legumes

- Raw nut butters

- Water

- Natural herbs and spices

- Seaweed

- Sprouted greens

- Superfoods

- Brown Rice and bulgar wheat

Foods that you can eat in moderation on the anti-inflammatory diet include:

- Roasted nuts and seeds – walnuts and almonds are rich in omega 3

- Soy based foods

- Dark chocolate – however, not all chocolate is beneficial. Ensure that the percentage contents are over 70% cacao.

- Roasted nut butters (not peanut!)

- Non-sprouted grain

- Salad dressing

- Dried fruit with added sulfites and sugar

Tips to Make the Anti-Inflammatory Diet Work for You

When it comes to the anti-inflammatory diet, there are a few things that you can do to help to make sure that your new diet is successful.

- Variety! Eating more variety can not only help you to avoid becoming bored with your diet, but it can also help you to get more nutrient variety in your diet.

- Eat fresh food! Fresh foods are the best foods for providing the nutrients that your body needs and VERY FEW naturally occurring foods are inflammatory.

- Avoid fast foods and processed foods! Processed foods and fast foods are loaded with preservatives and chemicals that your body has no idea what to do with. These elements prompt an inflammatory response in your body and should be avoided.

- Snack on fruits and vegetables. We all snack, but fruits and vegetables are nature's perfect snack foods!

- Know your calorie intake requirements. Even though the anti-inflammatory diet focuses on reducing inflammation, it is also important to monitor calorie intake to avoid excessive calories. Excessive calorie intake can lead to obesity which also results in inflammation within the body.

- Focus your diet on a healthy ratio of 40% carbohydrates, 30% fats, and 30% proteins. Make sure to include each of these food groups in to your meals.

Your saturated fat intake should not exceed more than 10% of your daily calorie intake. Saturated fats consist of animal fats such as cream, butter, and cheese. Avoid trans fats completely which include products like doughnuts, cakes, and many of the processed foods available.

- Include exercise in to your daily routine. Exercise tailored to your health level can help your body to produce natural anti-inflammatories that regulate current levels of inflammation and also help to prevent future inflammation.

Chapter 4: An Anti-Inflammatory Diet 7 Day Meal Plan

In the previous chapters we have covered a lot of the basics that you need to know about the anti-inflammatory diet. In this section we have a seven day menu on the anti-inflammatory diet. The recipes included in this menu will be covered in the following chapters.

The Menu

Monday

Breakfast: Organic mixed berries

Snack: Hardboiled omega-3 enriched egg

Lunch: Curried hummus and whole-grain pita

Snack: Grapefruit

Dinner: White chili

Snack: Fresh pineapple rings

Tuesday

Breakfast: Anti-inflammatory porridge

Snack: Celery sticks, raw broccoli and cauliflower with nut butter or leftover curried hummus

Lunch: Mixed greens salad with bell peppers, cucumber, carrots and hardboiled egg

Snack: Large orange

Dinner: Balsamic vinaigrette chicken with side salad

Snack: Whole baked sweet potato with cinnamon

Wednesday

Breakfast: Fresh raspberry smoothie

Snack: Almonds

Lunch: Bell pepper tuna salad

Snack: Halved avocado filled with fresh crab meat

Dinner: Fettuccini and pesto

Snack: Cantaloupe

Thursday

Breakfast: Rhubarb and ginger muffins

Snack: Citrus salad mix (orange, pineapple, and grapefruit cubed)

Lunch: Sweet potato soup

Snack: Low fat yogurt with fresh blueberries

Dinner: Lemon salmon with zucchini

Snack: Mixed raw nuts

Friday

Breakfast: Sweet potato frittata

Snack: Celery sticks with nut butter

Lunch: Chickpea salad

Snack: Thinly sliced salmon on whole wheat crackers

Dinner: Turkey stuffed bell peppers

Snack: Tropical fruit salad (papaya, nectarine, kiwi)

Saturday

Breakfast: Eggs in avocado

Snack: Edamame

Lunch: Quinoa, cashew salad

Snack: ½ cup applesauce mixed with ½ cup cottage cheese

Dinner: Red lentil and chard soup

Snack: Jarlsberg cheese with whole grain crackers and grapes

Sunday

Breakfast: Apple pie oatmeal

Snack: Cottage cheese with berries

Lunch: Black bean fried rice

Snack: Fresh shrimp and cocktail sauce

Dinner: Anti-inflammatory casserole

Snack: Apple sauce with cinnamon

Chapter 5: Anti-Inflammatory Breakfast Recipes

An important meal to get you started for the day, breakfast is the perfect chance to get started on the right foot. These breakfast recipes that were mentioned in chapter 4, are tasty, healthy, and filled with anti-inflammatory ingredients!

Breakfast Recipes

Anti-inflammatory porridge
Servings: 1

Ingredients:

- 1 ½ cups of rolled oats

- 3 ½ cups coconut milk

- 4 tbsp. chia seeds

- 3 tbsp. raw cacao

- 1 pinch of Stevia (a plant extract sweetener)

- Unsweetened coconut flakes to taste

- Fresh cherries to taste

- 1 pinch dark chocolate shavings

- Maple syrup to taste

Instructions:

In a large saucepan, combine your coconut milk, coats, cacao, and Stevia. Stir these ingredients to combine them thoroughly and heat over medium heat until it comes to a boil.

Once your ingredients are boiling, turn your heat down to low and let them simmer until your oats are cooked all the way through.

Once your oats are cooked through, put your porridge in to a serving bowl and garnish with your cherries, coconut shavings, dark chocolate, and maple syrup. Keep these toppings in moderation!

Fresh raspberry smoothie

Servings: 1

Calories: Unavailable

Fat: Unavailable

Protein: Unavailable

Net Carbs: Unavailable

Ingredients:

- 1 peeled and pitted avocado
- ¾ cup freshly squeezed orange juice
- ¾ cup raspberry juice (crush your raspberries to release the juice)
- ½ cup fresh raspberries

Instructions:

In a blender, combine all of your ingredients and puree until you get a smooth smoothie texture. If you need more liquid in your smoothie, add in a little water, ice or coconut milk.

Rhubarb and Ginger Muffins

Servings: 8

Ingredients:

- ½ cup almond meal
- ¼ cup unrefined raw sugar
- 2 tbsp. chopped crystallized ginger
- 1 tbsp. linseed meal
- ½ cup buckwheat flour
- ¼ cup fine brown rice flour
- 2 tbsp. organic corn flour
- 2 tsp. gluten-free baking powder
- ½ tsp. cinnamon
- ½ tsp. ground ginger
- 1 pinch sea salt
- 1 cup thinly sliced rhubarb
- 1 cored, peeled, diced apple
- 1/3 cup and 1 tbsp. almond milk
- ¼ cup olive oil
- 1 egg
- 1 tsp. vanilla extract

Instructions:

Begin by pre-heating your oven to 350 degrees.

While your oven pre-heats, line eight cups in a muffin pan and grease the cups, if needed using spray butter.

Now, take a medium mixing bowl and combine your ginger, almond meal, sugar, linseed meal, and ginger. Mix these ingredients together to combine.

Next, take a sieve, and sieve your baking powder, flours, and spices over this bowl of ingredients. Stir again to combine thoroughly. Add in your rhubarb and apple and mix until your rhubarb and apple are completely coated.

In a new mixing bowl, combine your egg, milk, oil, and vanilla extract and whisk them together well. Once mixed, add them to your larger bowl of mixed ingredients and stir until only just combined.

Divide your mixture of ingredients between your eight muffin cups and bake in the pre-heated oven for 20 minutes or until done all the way through.

Once cooked, remove your muffins from the oven and allow them to cool for a few minutes before setting them out on a cooling rack to cool completely.

Sweet Potato Soup

Servings: 6

Ingredients:

- 1 jar (12 oz.) roasted red peppers chopped (reserve juice)
- 2 chopped onions
- 4 cups peeled, cubed sweet potatoes
- 1 can (4 oz.) diced green chilies
- 2 tbsp. olive oil
- 2 tsp. cumin
- 1 tsp. salt
- 1 tsp. coriander
- 4 cups low-sodium vegetable broth
- 2 tbsp. fresh minced cilantro
- 1 tbsp. fresh lemon juice
- 4 oz. cream cheese cubed

Instructions:

Add your olive oil to a large soup pot and heat on your stovetop over high heat. Once hot, add in your onions and cook them until transparent. Then add in your red pepper, cumin, green chilies, coriander, and salt. Stir to combine and then cook for 2 minutes.

After 2 minutes, add in the juice from your red peppers along with your vegetable broth and your sweet potatoes. Stir gain and allow your ingredients to come to a boil.

Once your ingredients are boiling, turn down your heat to medium and cover the pot. Allow to cook for around 15 minutes or until your sweet potatoes are cooked through and tender. When tender, take your pot off the heat and add in your lemon juice and your cilantro and let the soup cool just a little.

Once slightly cooled, add your cream cheese in to your soup pot and use an immersion blender to smooth your soup out. Test your soup for temperature, and if needed heat a little more.

Taste your soup for seasoning and if required simply add a little more salt to taste before serving.

Sweet Potato Frittata

Servings: 2

Ingredients:

- 1 sweet potato
- 1 tbsp. olive oil
- 1 peeled, minced shallot
- Salt and pepper to taste
- 4 eggs
- 1 handful diced chives
- 8 oz. plum tomatoes
- 2 trimmed, sliced green onions
- 1 handful chopped cilantro
- ½ lemon for juice
- 3 tbsp. olive oil
- 1 tbsp. sesame oil
- 1 dash Tabasco

Instructions:

Begin by preparing your salsa. Cut your tomatoes in to quarters and add them to a medium sized mixing bowl. Add in your green onions, cilantro, lemon juice, 3 tbsp. olive oil, 1 tbsp. sesame oil, and tabasco sauce. Mix these ingredients together to combine them well and taste. If desired add salt and pepper.

Now set your broiler to its highest heat. While it heats, peel your sweet potato and cut in to small cubes.

Next, take a large broiler proof skillet or pan and heat your olive oil on medium heat. Once your oil is hot throw in your sweet potato and your shallot. Season lightly with salt and pepper and stir. Cook while stirring occasionally for around 5 minutes or until your potatoes are lightly browned and only just tender.

While your sweet potatoes brown, take a medium sized mixing bowl and beat your eggs with your chives. Once they are well beaten, pour your egg mixture over the browned sweet potatoes. Make sure that your ingredients are all well distributed through the pan. Turn your heat down to low.

Let your frittata cook on low heat (don't stir!) so that your egg begins to firm a little. Now, take your pan and put it under your broiler just until the top of your frittata is completely set. Make sure not to overcook your frittata!

Once your eggs are set, take your pan out of the oven and use a spatula to flip your frittata out on to your plate.

Top your frittata with your salsa mixture and serve!

Eggs in Avocado

Servings: 1

Ingredients:

- 2 eggs
- 1 ripe avocado halved
- Salt and pepper to taste
- 1 tbsp. fresh chives chopped

Instructions:

If you haven't already, half your avocado and remove the pit.

Set your oven to pre-heat to 425 degrees.

While your oven heats, take a baking dish and place your avocados in to it with the open side facing upwards. You may need to place the avocado halves at the sides of the dish so that they lean against it.

Now, crack one egg in to the center of each avocado.

Once your oven has pre-heated, bake your avocado in the oven for 15 to 20 minutes or until your egg has set fully.

Once cooked, take your baking dish out of the oven and season your eggs and avocados with salt and pepper. Garnish the tops of your avocados with your chives and serve!

Apple Pie Oatmeal
Servings: 4

Ingredients:

- 3 cups filtered water
- ¾ steel cut oats
- 2 tsp. pumpkin pie spice
- 70g protein powder
- 1 cup unsweetened apple sauce
- 1 tsp. Stevia extract
- 16 pecan halves

Instructions:

In a large saucepan, bring your water to a boil. Once boiling, mix in your oats as well as your pumpkin pie spice. Stir well to combine your ingredients in the water and then allow this mixture to cook for 5 minutes.

After 5 minutes, turn your heat down to a simmer and let simmer for 30 minutes.

Once 30 minutes have passed, take your pan off the heat and set your oats aside to allow them to cool.

When your oats have fully cooled, stir your protein powder in to them.

If you are ready to eat right away, stir in the rest of your ingredients and serve! If you want to eat this warm, just put it in the microwave 30 seconds at a time, stirring between each 30 second interval.

Chapter 6: Anti-Inflammatory Lunch Recipes

In this chapter we will include recipes for the lunchtime anti-inflammatory meals included in our 7-day dietary plan. These recipes include plenty of variation and are light enough to be filling, and not so heavy that they weigh you down for the rest of the day.

Lunch Recipes

Curried Hummus
Servings: 16

Ingredients:

- 2 cans (15 ½ oz.) drained and rinsed garbanzo beans

- 3 crushed garlic cloves

- 2 tbsp. olive oil

- 6 tbsp. fresh organic lemon juice

- 4 tsp. curry powder

- ½ cup filtered water

- Hot sauce to taste

- Salt to taste

Instructions:

Throw all of your ingredients in to your food processor and blend them together until you get a smooth hummus-like consistency. Scoop your hummus out in to a bowl and if you like you can drizzle the top of it with olive oil before serving. It is recommended to serve this hummus with multi-grain pitas.

Bell pepper tuna salad

Servings: 2

Ingredients:

- 2 stemmed, ribbed, seeded red bell peppers with just the tops cut off
- 2 drained cans (5 oz.) tuna in water
- ¼ cup chopped olives
- ¼ cup mayonnaise
- 2 tbsp. minced red onion
- 2 tbsp. chopped roasted red peppers
- 2 tbsp. fresh chopped basil
- 1 tbsp. capers
- 1 tbsp. freshly squeezed lemon juice
- Salt and pepper to taste

Instructions:

In a large mixing bowl, combine all of your ingredients except for your bell peppers. With a large mixing spoon, combine these ingredients to mix them well.

Now take two small plates and stand up your red peppers on their bottoms on each plate. Now divide your tuna salad between the two peppers and spoon it inside.

Carefully use a knife to slice off the excess pepper at the top of each pepper. Slice this removed pepper in to slices and use these to dip in to the tuna salad. Serve.

Chickpea Salad
Servings: 4

Ingredients:

- 2 cans (19 oz.) drained and rinsed chickpeas
- 1 grated carrot
- ½ diced red onion
- ½ diced green bell pepper
- ¼ cup fresh lemon juice
- 2 tbsp. olive oil
- Salt and pepper to taste
- ¼ cup chopped fresh parsley leaves

Instructions:

In a large mixing bowl, combine all of your ingredients and toss to ensure that they are distributed evenly. Serve in a small bowl. If desired, accompany with fresh sliced vegetables.

Quinoa, Cashew Salad

Servings: 4

Ingredients:

- 1 cup rinsed quinoa
- ½ red onion chopped
- 1 cup chopped apple
- 1 lime for juice
- 2 tbsp. honey
- 1 tbsp. olive oil
- 1 chopped mango (firmer ripe rather than softer ripe)
- ¼ cup chopped fresh mint leaves
- 1 tsp. sea salt
- Black pepper to taste
- ½ inch knob ginger chopped
- 1 sliced avocado
- 1 cup chopped cashews
- 3 cups chopped romaine lettuce

Instructions:

Begin by boiling 2 cups of water on your stovetop over medium-high heat.

Once boiling, take your quinoa and add to the pan of water. Turn down your heat on your pan to maintain a simmer and cover your pan. Let your quinoa simmer for 20 minutes to cook thoroughly.

Once your quinoa is cooked through, set it aside to allow it to cool.

While your quinoa cools, take a large mixing bowl and combine your apple and red onion together. Use your hands to toss these together to mix them thoroughly.

Now, take a small bowl and mix together your honey, lime juice, and olive oil. Whisk to mix well. Once mixed, add to your apple and red onion mixture. Now add in your cooled quinoa as well as your mango. Use salad tongs or your hands to mix these ingredients together thoroughly.

Next, add in your mint, ginger, cilantro, and a little salt and pepper to taste and lightly toss your ingredients together to mix your spices throughout.

Now, put out your greens on to serving plates or dishes and spoon your mixture from your bowl on top of your greens. Top the plate with your avocado slices and sprinkle with your cashews.

If desired, chill the salad before serving or serve on chilled plates, but this salad can be served at room temperature as well.

Black Bean Fried Rice

Servings: 4

Ingredients:

- 2 tbsp. coconut oil
- 2 diced carrots
- 1 diced onion
- 1 bunch sliced scallions
- 1 cup sliced snap peas
- 2 minced garlic cloves
- 1 tbsp. fresh minced ginger
- 3 cups cooked black rice
- 3 tbsp. liquid aminos
- 2 tsp. toasted sesame oil
- 1 tsp. Sriracha
- 2 beaten eggs
- 1 tbsp. shelled hemp seed

Instructions:

Take a large skillet and heat your coconut oil over medium-high heat. Once your oil is hot, add in your onion, carrot and white scallion pieces and sauté until they begin to brown. Next, add in your ginger, snap peas, garlic, and green scallion pieces to the skillet and stir to distribute. Once well mixed, allow this mixture to cook for 2 minutes.

After 2 minutes, you want to stir in your black rice and continue to cook for 2 minutes. Continue folding your rice mixture as the rice starts to toast. After your rice has toasted and your 2 minutes are up, add your sesame oil, Sriracha, and liquid aminos. Stir once again to disburse.

Now, use a spatula or cooking spoon and more your rice mixture over to one side of your pan. Next, pour your eggs in to the middle of the pan and cook until they are almost firmed. Now toss them with the rice mixture and the hemp seeds and plate in serving bowls to serve!

Chapter 7: Anti-Inflammatory Dinner Recipes

In this chapter we cover the dinner recipes included in our 7-day sample menu in chapter 4. These recipes are healthy but filling and a great way to take advantage of inflammation reducing foods.

Dinner Recipes

White Chili
Servings: 8-10

Ingredients:

- 1lb. skinless, boneless chicken breast

- 1 diced onion

- 2 tbsp. extra virgin olive oil

- 2 minced garlic cloves

- 1 cup fresh corn

- 2 cans (15 oz.) drained, rinsed white beans

- 1 can (4 oz.) chopped green chilies

- 2 tsp. cumin

- 2 tsp. chili powder

- 1/8 tsp. cayenne pepper

- 3 cups filtered water

- 2 cups grated Monterey Jack

- 2 tbsp. chopped cilantro

Instructions:

Take your chicken breasts and season them with salt and pepper and set them aside.

Now, heat your olive oil over high heat in a large pan. Once heated, cook your pieces of chicken until they are browned on both sides.

When your chicken is browned, turn down your heat to medium and throw in your garlic and onion. Stir to mix these ingredients and allow them to cook until your onion is clear.

Once your onion is clear, throw your corn, beans, water, and your spices and mix well to combine. Now turn your heat down to low and allow your pan to simmer for an hour without covering it.

After an hour of simmering, plate your chili and garnish with your cheese and cilantro.

Balsamic Vinaigrette Chicken

Servings: 4

Ingredients:

- 1 pieced out (4 lb.) whole chicken
- ¼ cup balsamic vinegar
- 2 tbsp. Dijon mustard
- 2 tbsp. fresh lemon juice
- 2 tbsp. olive oil
- 2 chopped garlic cloves
- Salt and pepper to taste
- ½ cup low-sodium chicken broth
- 1 tsp. lemon zest
- 1 tbsp. fresh chopped parsley

Instructions:

In a small mixing bowl, combine your mustard, garlic, vinegar, lemon juice, olive oil, salt and pepper. Whisk these ingredients together well to combine.

Now, take a large freezer bag and pour your whisked ingredients in to the bag and put your chicken in to the bag. Close the bag and make sure that your chicken is coated thoroughly in the dressing mix. Now put your bag in to the refrigerator for at least two hours. You can refrigerate your chicken for as long as 24 hours.

After your chicken has been marinated, pre-heat your oven to 400 degrees. While your oven pre-heats, take out a baking dish and grease using cooking spray. Set out your chicken pieces in your dish.

When the oven is pre-heated, put your baking dish in to the oven and bake your chicken for around 60 minutes, or until your chicken is cooked all the way through.

Once your chicken is cooked through, put it on to a serving plate. Now pour your drippings in to a small saucepan and put on the stove on medium-low heat. Use a whisk to mix in your chicken broth, making sure to scrape up any of the bits that have stuck to the bottom of the pan. Once the broth mixture is heated all the way through, use a spoon to drizzle it over your chicken on the serving plate.

When ready to serve, top your chicken with your lemon zest and parsley.

Fettuccini and Pesto

Servings: 1

Ingredients:

- ¼ lb. whole grain fettuccine pasta
- ¼ cup grated parmigiana-reggiano cheese
- 1 cup stemmed chopped kale (for your pesto)
- 1/8 cup grated parmigiana-reggiano (for your pesto)
- 1 ½ tbsp. extra virgin olive oil (for your pesto)
- 1/16 cup pine nuts (for your pesto)
- ½ chopped garlic clove (for your pesto)
- ¼ tsp. salt (for your pesto)
- 1 pinch red pepper flakes (for your pesto)

Instructions:

Begin by starting your pasta cooking.

Now, while your pasta is cooking, take your food processor, combine your pesto ingredients and mix thoroughly until you get a pesto like consistency.

When your pasta is fully cooked, plate it and mix in your pesto mixture and mix well before serving!

Lemon Salmon with Zucchini

Servings: 4

Ingredients:

- 4 chopped zucchini
- 2 tbsp. olive oil
- Salt and pepper to taste
- 2 tbsp. packed brown sugar
- 2 tbsp. freshly squeezed lemon juice
- 1 tbsp. Dijon mustard
- 2 minced garlic cloves
- ½ tsp. dried dill
- ½ tsp. dried oregano
- ¼ tsp. dried thyme
- ¼ tsp. dried rosemary
- 4 (5-ounce each) salmon fillets
- 2 tbsp. fresh chopped parsley

Instructions:

Begin by pre-heating your oven to 400 degrees. While your oven pre-heats, take a baking tray and cover it with aluminum foil. Grease your foil with non-stick butter.

Now, take a mixing bowl and combine your Dijon, brown sugar, lemon juice, dill, garlic, thyme, oregano, and rosemary. Season lightly with your salt and pepper and mix thoroughly to combine.

Next, set your zucchini out on your baking tray and sprinkle with olive oil. Season lightly with salt and pepper. Add your salmon to the tray as well and brush your herb mix from the mixing bowl over your salmon.

When your oven is pre-heated, bake your salmon and zucchini in the oven for around 16 minutes or until your fish is flakey.

Serve your salmon and zucchini as soon as it comes out of the oven.

Turkey Stuffed Bell Peppers

Servings: 3

Ingredients:

- 3 yellow bell peppers
- 1 ¼ lb. lean ground turkey
- 1 cup diced mushrooms
- ¼ cup diced onion
- 1 cup chopped fresh spinach
- 2 tsp. minced garlic
- 1 cup tomato sauce
- 1 cup low-sodium chicken broth
- 1 cup dried quinoa

Instructions:

Begin by cooking your quinoa in a saucepan according to the directions on the packet.

While your quinoa cooks, heat some olive oil in a skillet over medium-high heat. Once hot, throw your vegetables (not your yellow pepper) in to the pan and sauté for 5 minutes.

After 5 minutes, add your garlic and ground turkey in to your skillet, stir and cook on medium heat. Continue to cook until your turkey is almost completely cooked through and then add in half of your chicken broth and your tomato sauce. Stir your ingredients to combine and then let them simmer until your turkey is cooked through. At this point you should have some of the extra liquid in your pan cooked off as well.

Pre-heat your oven to 400 degrees.

While your turkey mix is still cooking, wash your bell peppers and slice them in half vertically. Take out the stems, seeds and ribs.

Take out a 9" x 13" baking pan and spray with spray butter. Now set your bell peppers in to the pan with the open side up.

When your quinoa has completely cooked, add it to the pan of your turkey mixture and mix to combine. Once well mixed, divide the mixture between each half of your bell peppers and fill them.

Take the rest of your chicken broth and pour it in to the bottom of your baking pan and cover the pan with aluminum foil. Bake your stuffed peppers for 30 minutes and serve warm!

Red Lentil and Chard Soup

Servings: 4

Ingredients:

- 1 diced onion
- 2 diced carrots
- 2 minced garlic cloves
- 2 tbsp. olive oil
- 1 tsp. cumin
- ½ tsp. ground ginger
- ½ tsp. ground turmeric
- ½ tsp. red chili flakes
- ½ tsp. sea salt
- 1 can (15 oz.) diced tomatoes
- 1 cup dried split red lentils
- 2 quarts low-sodium vegetable stock
- 1 bunch stemmed, chopped chard

Instructions:

In a large soup pot, add your oil and heat over medium-high heat.

Once your oil is heated, throw your carrot and onion in to the pot and cook until your carrot is tender and your onion is starting to brown. Once this happens, add your ginger, garlic, cumin, chili flakes, turmeric, and salt in to the pot and stir to mix thoroughly. Cook for just a minute before adding in your tomatoes.

Stir your pot after adding in your tomatoes, making sure to scrape up any browned pieces that have stuck to the bottom of the pot. Allow this mixture to cook until your liquid has almost cooked off and your tomatoes have softened.

Once your tomatoes are soft, add your stock as well as your lentils to the soup pan and allow the ingredients to come to a boil. Once boiling, turn your heat down to allow your mixture to simmer. Let your pot simmer for as long as it takes for your lentils to soften – this should be around 10 minutes.

When your lentils have softened, fold in your chard and allow it to cook for just a few minutes so that your chard is wilted but not soggy.

Taste your soup to ensure it needs no more seasoning. If needed, add more seasoning to your taste.

Plate your soup, and serve with a small wedge of lemon for garnish.

Anti-Inflammatory Casserole

Servings: 6

Ingredients:

- 4 ½ cups whole wheat pasta
- 1 tbsp. olive oil
- 5 oz. lean ground turkey
- 4 chopped Roma tomatoes
- 1 cup chopped red bell pepper
- 1 ½ cups chopped onion
- 16 oz. fresh green beans
- 26 oz. tomato sauce
- 1 cup filtered water
- 1 tsp. Italian seasoning
- 1 tsp. dried basil
- Salt and pepper to taste
- ¾ cup shredded part-skim mozzarella
- 1 ½ tbsp. olive oil for drizzling

Instructions:

Begin by pre-heating your oven to 350 degrees.

While your oven pre-heats, take out a baking dish that measures 13" x 9" and spray it with non-stick cooking spray. Set this dish aside for the moment.

Now, take a large skillet and over medium-high heat bring your olive oil up to temperature. Once hot, add your turkey, onion and bell pepper to the skillet and mix thoroughly. Allow this mixture to cook until your turkey is browned.

When your turkey is cooked through, add your green beans, water, tomato sauce, spices, pasta, and salt and pepper. Mix these ingredients thoroughly to combine them and allow the mixture to cook for around 10 to 15 minutes until your pasta is cooked all the way through.

Once your pasta is cooked, take your skillet off the heat and spoon your mixture in to your casserole dish. Put the dish in to your pre-heated oven and cook for 25 minutes.

After 25 minutes, take your casserole dish out of the oven and top it with your cheese. After topping the casserole with cheese, put your dish in to the oven and bake without a cover for between 5 to 10 minutes. By this time the cheese on top of your casserole should have melted and browned.

Take your thoroughly cooked casserole out of the oven and slice. Plate each portion and then drizzle each portion with olive oil before serving.

Chapter 8: Shopping list

Vegetables
- Asparagus, Arugula, Beets, Bell Peppers, Broccoli, Brussels Sprouts, Bok Choi, Cabbage, Cauliflower, Carrots, Celery, Corn, Cucumber, Fennel, Green Beans, Kale, Lettuce, Mushroom, Onions, Peas, Potatoes, Pumpkin, Radishes, Spinach, Squash, Sweet Potatoes, Swiss Chard, Tomatoes, Turnips

Fruits
- Apples, Apricots, Avocados, Bananas, Blueberries, Cherries, Cranberries, Prunes, Figs, Grapefruit, Grapes, Kiwis, Lemons and Limes, Mangoes, Oranges, Papaya, Peaches, Pineapple, Plums Raisons, Raspberries, Strawberries, Watermelon

Fish
- Cod, Halibut, Mackerel, Mussels, Oyster, Salmon, Scallops, Shrimp, Tuna

Grains
- Amaranth, Barley, Brown Rice, Bulgar, Farro, Millet, Oatmeal, Quinoa, Wheat berries, Whole Wheat Pasta, Whole Grain Breads

Herbs/Spices
- Allspice, Basil, Bay Leaf, Chervil, Chives, Cinnamon, Clove, Dill, Garlic, Ginger, Mustard, Nutmeg, Paprika, Parsley, Pepper, Peppermint, Rosemary, Saffron, Sage, Tarragon, Thyme

Legumes/Nuts/Seeds
- Almonds, Black Beans, Chickpeas, Flax, Kidney Beans, Lentils, Peanut Butter, Pine nuts, Pinto beans, Pistachios, Pumpkins Seeds, Sesame Seeds, Soybeans, Sunflower Seeds, Tofu, Walnuts

Oils
- Safflower Oil, Sunflower oil, Extra Virgin Olive Oil

Conclusion

I hope this book was able to help you to understand how your body is affected by inflammation, as well as how you can control the symptoms through your diet. By following the information provided in the chapters above I am certain that you will see positive changes in your overall health.

So, where do you go from here? The first step is making a full commitment to a lifestyle change – this means going through your pantry and eliminating those inflammatory foods. From there it's up to you to make better eating choices using the guidelines provided. They may seem difficult at first, but when you consider that it's your health and a lifetime of possible disability on the line, it really isn't that hard!

Finally, if you have an interest in other diets to help with weight loss and a healthier lifestyle please check out my others books available on Amazon.

Paleo Diet - The Essential Paleo Guide For Rapid Weight Loss And Healthy Living - Includes 36 Delicious Recipes For Every Meal – John Richards

Atkins Diet - The Complete Atkins Diet Guide And Low Carb Recipe Plan For Permanent Weight Loss And Optimum Health – Includes 36 low carb recipes – John Richards

Ketogenic Diet: The Ultimate Low Carb Diet And Recipe Plan For Rapid Weight Loss And Healthy Living - Includes 7 Day Meal Plan With Over 20 Ketogenic Recipes – John Richards

Made in the USA
Middletown, DE
26 May 2016